morning

TOP TIPS FOR A HEALTHIER FUTURE

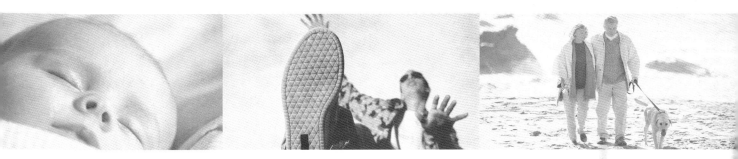

CONTENTS

page	
2	Making the best of your doctor and your prescriptions
4	Planning pregnancy
5	When you can't get pregnant
6	After the birth
7	Looking after yourself
8	Your growing baby
9	Terrible twos
10	Coughs and colds all the time
11	Help! My toddler won't sleep
12	Asthma
14	When to go to the doctor
15	Growing up
17	Drug taking in teenagers
18	Teenagers and stress
19	Stress
20	Breast lumps
21	Breast cancer
22	Back pain
23	Snoring

page	
24	Irritable bowel syndrome
25	Ulcers
26	Period problems
28	Weight management
29	Smoking
30	Blood pressure
31	Heart health for women
32	Menopause
33	Hormone replacement therapy
34	Osteoporosis
36	Diabetes
38	Arthritis
40	Replacement hip
42	Prostate problems
43	Caring for someone who is confused
45	Travel
46	Sun
47	Coping with an emergency
48	Further information and advice

MAKING THE BEST OF YOUR DOCTOR AND YOUR PRESCRIPTIONS

How to choose a doctor Ask around, particularly parents of young children.

Go to the local library – each local practice supplies them with a practice leaflet, which shows things like the ages and sex of their doctors which may help you decide if what you'd like is an older woman doctor.

Alternatively ask for details from the Regional health information service on 0800 66 55 44.

Changing doctors If you don't have confidence in your GP, or don't like him or her, change doctors but preferably at a time when you're relaxed, rather than in the middle of a crisis. You can also phone the number above for advice.

If you don't have an alternative, because you live in a small town, ask to be assigned to a different partner in the practice.

Make a friend of the receptionist They're not always the dragons they're made out to be and are definitely worth cultivating.

Remember, the receptionist is your gateway to the doctor, so don't get cross with them.

When you're with the doctor Be honest.

Tell him everything – for instance if you have two symptoms, don't just tell him the one you think is the most important, tell him both. It may help his diagnosis.

Be clear about time – when did you first notice your symptoms, when did they change?

If your mind tends to go blank, write down the questions you want to ask.

Don't be embarrassed – they've seen it all before!

What annoys doctors?
Patients who say they're desperate to see you who then don't turn up.

People who ask you for your opinion about someone else's illness.

People who grab you in the supermarket car park when you're doing the shopping with the family and want a diagnosis.

People who lie to you about how much they're smoking or drinking.

People who don't take medicines that you know would help them.

People who want everything done now – like all the travel jabs the day before they go.

Worst of all?
'Not annoying, heartbreaking – people who don't tell you about their symptoms because they don't want to bother you, and who only tell you when it's too late to help them'.

Helping the medicine do its job Three out of four people will be prescribed medicines when they visit their GPs. Because there may be so much else to take in at the time, you may forget to ask your doctor about your medicine. But your questions can often make a big difference to how well the medicine works for you. Here are the most important ones.

Why is your doctor giving it to you and what does he think it will do for you?

What is it called? Drug names can be very confusing as most have at least two – a chemical name and one or more brand names. Ask for both.

What's the dose? Tip: if the dose is 'a teaspoon', ask for a 5ml spoon from the pharmacist. You can overdose if you use home teaspoons which may hold twice as much.

How often should I take it? Four times a day usually means at four equal intervals during waking hours – first thing, lunchtime, teatime and bedtime – not at 8 am, 2 pm, 8 pm, 2 am but check. Try to take your medicine at the recommended interval – taking doses too close together increases the risk of medicine side-effects.

How long should I carry on taking it? Even though you may be feeling better, you still need to carry on taking medicines such as antibiotics until the course is finished.

Any special instructions? For instance, not to take milk or indigestion remedies at the same time as the medicine (it may mean it won't work properly). Alcohol is best avoided with many drugs. Ask whether you should take your medicine with or without food. Should you still drive? Will they affect your work?

Will there be any side effects? Not everyone will get them but if you do, most will lessen as your body gets used to the medicine. If they persist, it may be possible to alter the dose or change drugs. But don't just stop taking your medicine as this in itself may cause problems. If you are worried, check with your doctor.

Can I take it with my other medicines? Always mention what other medicines you are taking as some drugs interact, making them less effective or causing other problems.

How soon before I feel better? Some drugs work quickly but it may be several weeks before you notice the beneficial effects of others such as anti-depressants.

YOU THE EXPERT

'Taking lots of tablets got me really confused. Then I got a tablet dispenser from my local chemist – there are several little compartments for each day and now I can see at a glance exactly what I need to take.'
Mrs E Mills, Hove

TOP TIPS

- shake the bottle (the active ingredient may have settled at the bottom)

- take tablets with water, when sitting or standing, never when lying down as this may lead to choking

- a drink of cold water immediately after nasty medicine hides the taste

If you're thinking about starting a family, now is the time to reconsider your lifestyle – not just because you want a baby but because your good health practices will become those of your children, not just for their childhood but for life.

Although there can never be any guarantees, being healthy yourself makes it more likely that your baby will be healthy too.

Get fit! The more active and fit you are now, the easier you'll find it to cope with pregnancy – and get back into shape afterwards.

If you're overweight or underweight you'll find it harder to conceive. And being the right weight for your height when you fall pregnant is the single most important factor determining your baby's health at birth (see p. 28).

Stop smoking! Smoker's babies are more likely to be premature and to be born underweight. And smoker's children are more like to suffer from illnesses like asthma. Try to give it up now. If you find it hard, phone the smoker's Quitline on 0800 00 22 00.

Eat well! Try to make a conscious effort to improve the quality of your diet, with a good mixture of different foods, including at least five portions daily of fruit and vegetables.

Folic acid, a B vitamin, will protect your baby against spina bifida and other neural tube defects but only if taken in larger amounts than you're likely to get in your diet. So take one tablet daily of the right strength (400 mcg) as soon as you decide you want to start trying for a baby and for the first 12 weeks of pregnancy.

Cut down on alcohol! Excessive drinking can affect the baby's health and weight at birth, and getting drunk can be particularly risky. Women trying to get pregnant or at any stage of pregnancy should therefore avoid intoxication and drink no more than one or two units once or twice a week.

Ask your GP

- To check whether you are immune to rubella (German Measles) even if you have been immunised.

- For advice about possible changes to your medication if you are taking medicines regularly.

- For advice if you are epileptic, diabetic or have other chronic health conditions.

- For advice if you have had previous pregnancy problems such as the birth of a handicapped baby.

YOU THE EXPERT

'I know planning doesn't guarantee anything, but at least you avoid all that worry of discovering you're pregnant only after you've done all the wrong things.' Sally Brookes, Newcastle

At least one child in seven has asthma in the UK. Tobacco smok

From all you're told about contraception, you'd think getting pregnant was very easy. Actually, it takes the average British couple about six months to conceive. And it's normal for a quarter of all couples to take a year. A year may feel like a lifetime to you and you may become increasingly frustrated and disappointed when pregnancy doesn't happen. Even if sperm and egg meet and the earth moves, there is still only a 1 in 4 chance of pregnancy in any one cycle – and that's normal.

HOW TO WORK OUT YOUR FERTILE PERIOD

Keep a record of your periods over a few months.

Find out your longest and shortest cycle by counting from the day your period starts to the day the next one starts (e.g. 32 days and 27 days). Subtract 14 (the length of the second half of your cycle) from these numbers. Ovulation (the time of maximum fertility) is likely to occur between day 13 (27–14) and day 18 (32–14) of your current cycle.

What you can do for yourself Minimise pressure from friends and family and keep the fact you're planning pregnancy to yourselves.

Don't restrict your lovemaking to just once in your fertile period. It's too pressurising and your chances will be increased if you make love frequently (every two to three days) throughout your cycle.

Ask your man to cut down on heavy drinking and smoking (they affect sperm quantity and quality).

When to go to your GP and ask for help After 18 months of unprotected sex if you are 30 or under, after a year if you are over 30, or within a few months if you have had any of the following.

- if you have very irregular periods or have had recent very heavy periods (possible ovulation problems).
- if sex hurts and you have painful and or very heavy periods (possible endometriosis).
- you have a history of pelvic infection or burst appendix (possible tubal damage).
- if your partner has had testicular infection, injury or surgery, mumps in adult life or undescended testicles.

What will your GP do?

Offer a blood test to the woman to check whether she is ovulating.

Offer a simple sperm test to the man to check sperm numbers.

ncreases the risk of children with asthma having an attack.

Now what? For the last nine months you were the centre of attention, you probably looked and felt great, organised your home efficiently and held down a job as well. Yet here you are, stuck at home with a thing in a basket that cries all the time and makes constant demands on you. You're feeling exhausted, flabby, miserable and unable to get out of your dressing gown before lunchtime. Nobody ever said it would be like this.

In this situation, your GP and your midwife or health visitor can be your lifeline.

Crying Babies cry. Some of them cry a lot. Mostly this means there is something wrong – they might be hungry, have a dirty nappy, be too hot or cold, be tired but unable to sleep, have colic or wind or just be bored and want company. You may exhaust this list and still have a crying baby. All sorts of advice may be offered and you may end up feeling that you're no good as a mother.

How to cope

- don't blame yourself
- try not to let yourself be undermined by 'advice' from friends and relatives
- try to share the soothing of your baby with your partner, your mum or a friend
- rhythmic movement, like rocking or pram jiggling soothes most. Find out what suits your baby best when cheerful and use a combination of two when fretful
- get out of the house – visit friends or a mums and baby club
- if you feel it's all getting too much, phone CRY-SIS (see p. 48) who will put you in touch with parents who've been in the same situation

Sleeping problems It takes a while for babies to develop a routine of their own. By 3 months, most will be having their main sleep at night. But many babies are still up twice or more a night. They appear not to suffer – you and your partner are the ones who are wrecked.

- try to establish a bedtime routine, e.g. bath, story, feed, bed
- always put your baby to sleep in the same place when at home
- give him* a chance to settle
- don't rock him to sleep in your arms, put him in her cot whilst still awake

YOU THE EXPERT

'My baby screamed from 6 pm to 2 am every single day for 3 months. My husband insisted I do something for myself every day, even if it was only gossiping on the phone to a friend. It helped keep me sane.' Lise Wallis, Leicester

6

* For convenience, the male gender is used in this book although, of course, the problems and suggested solutions apply to both sexes.

Every year there are about 35

Coping Almost all new mothers complain of being tired. Lack of sleep, getting over the birth and a demanding baby is an exhausting cocktail for anyone, so try and get as much rest as you can. For a while you simply won't be able to do everything you did before as well as look after a baby, so don't try it.

- the housework can wait
- make yourself have a rest every day
- make meals simple
- try not to have too many visitors
- accept all the help that you're offered

Postnatal depression Where does mild depression – common in most new mothers in the first weeks after birth – end and postnatal depression (PND) begin? Is this you or someone you know?

- do you have strong feelings of being worthless or inadequate?
- find it difficult to complete even the simplest tasks?
- be good at caring for the baby, but avoid eye contact with it?
- have outbursts of irrational anger or weeping?
- feel very isolated, but still prefer to stay at home rather than meet other mums?

If this sounds very familiar, then help is needed urgently. Talk to your health visitor or GP or get in contact with the Association for Post-Natal Illness (see p. 48). PND doesn't affect a particular 'type' of person – it can affect anyone, with 'copers' often being hit worst.

Getting back in to shape Getting back in to shape after a baby may be harder than it seems. You may not have the same opportunities for exercise as you did before and many mums find they snack more if they are at home all day. Remember it took nine months to put that weight on, so don't expect overnight miracles.

- try a brisk walk every day with the pram
- do your pelvic floor exercises in odd moments during the day
- eat a balanced diet
- join a postnatal exercise class – you may find it's more motivating

000 first-time births in England.

Development reviews will be offered to you by your GP or health visitor on a regular basis. They're an opportunity to share any concerns you may have, not just the big things but everyday niggles too.

They're offered at 6–8 weeks, and again at 6–9 months old, but if you're worried about something at any other time, don't wait, ask to see someone. Problems with breastfeeding, weaning and sleeping are the most common.

Problems with breastfeeding Sore or cracked nipples, leaking at the most inopportune moments, and your partner can't do it for you. Why did you think breastfeeding was such a good idea? But if you persevere past the initial difficulties, breastfeeding is bliss and is much more beneficial for the baby. The golden rule is to have your baby correctly positioned, but without under breast wing mirrors, it's hard to tell whether you're getting it right. This is where a health professional's advice is invaluable. Here are some other tips.

- if you have a problem, such as lumpy or tender breasts, tell someone quickly before it gets out of hand
- don't restrict your baby's access to the breast

Starting your baby on solid food It's easy to be rushed into starting your baby on solid food before he is ready for it. As a guide, babies can't digest food other than milks until they're about 4 months old.

- try starting with vegetable or fruit purees or baby rice. A small spoonful is enough at first, offered after the middle milk feed of the day. Be prepared for your baby to spit it out. Offer the same food again another day, but don't persist if he doesn't like it
- don't give eggs, wheat based foods such as wheat cereals, cow's milk, citrus fruit, very fatty food, nuts or foods containing nuts as all these can upset your baby or trigger an allergy

What next?
- add solid food at another mealtime, then another
- you can sieve or puree your own food, but don't add salt or sugar when preparing it
- you should still avoid the list of foods just mentioned until the baby is at least six months old
- from between 6–9 months, your baby can have any food you have, providing it's mashed up. Offer fruit juice (diluted 1:5) or water to drink with meals. Don't use cow's milk as a drink by itself until your baby is more than 12 months old
- Iron is important for children of this age. It is most easily absorbed from meat, but it is also in pulses and green vegetables. Absorption is helped by eating fruit or vegetables and drinking diluted fruit juice with the meal.

There are more than 6 million visits

TERRIBLE TWOS

By now, you will have discovered that there is no reasoning with a toddler and in a battle of wills, your toddler has what it takes to win every time.

Temper tantrums Most toddlers have developed tantrums to an art form. They work best with an audience, which is why they so often occur in crowded supermarkets. Here are some tips.

- remember, tantrums are a passing phase, not a pattern for life
- diversions as the tantrum gathers steam work well as in, at the crucial moment 'Good heavens, there's a monkey in our garden'.
- ignoring works well, as long as you can keep a cool exterior
- when you both threaten to go ballistic, firmly and coolly, take your shrieking toddler to his bedroom and leave him there, whilst you beat a swift retreat. This is not a punishment – just a means of separating you and allowing all parties to cool off.

Eating problems When your baby was little, you may have felt rather smug: 'My baby eats anything' you might have told your friends. As babies reach the toddler stage, all that changes. Your toddler may refuse everything except chicken nuggets and chocolate buttons. Suddenly mealtimes are battlegrounds. Do not waste your time trying to argue with a two year old about vitamins and health. Within reason, give him what food he wants, when he wants it and when he's hungry. Once he's learned to like food, then you can fight over eating it at the proper time. If your toddler has lots of energy, don't fret over how little food he is eating.

- remember many easily prepared foods are still nutritious – including baked beans, nuggets, etc.
- if your child won't eat a variety of foods, better to give him what he will eat
- increase variety by making nutritious 'snacks' to munch on between meals
- don't spend hours cooking – it's even harder to stay calm if it's not eaten
- if he doesn't eat at meals, don't let him fill up with sweets, biscuits and soft drinks etc. between meals

YOU THE EXPERT

'My toddler was a shocker for eating. So, we had 'picnics'. It was the same food, but just put in little boxes and transported somewhere else. He wolfed it down.' Sally Rogers, Kingston

If you're an adult and only get a couple of colds a year, it can be quite a worry when your child has one cold after another. You have developed some measure of immunity – but your child is prey to every new virus splattered on him by well meaning playmates. Once they start playgroup, average toddlers get up to nine colds a year with six being the usual number.

You can't prevent your child getting colds but you can do something about smoking. Every year 17,000 children are admitted to hospital because their parents smoke. Smoker's children are more likely to get coughs and colds, chest infections, ear infections and asthma.

Colds

- colds – are caused by viruses so antibiotics won't help
- break open one of those capsules containing decongestants on your child's pillow – it may help with breathing

Coughs

- most are caused by viruses. If the cough is bad and won't go away see your GP
- if the cough seems more troublesome at night or is brought on when your child is active, or if your child seems wheezy or breathless, she may have asthma and needs to be seen and assessed by your GP (see p.12)

Croup

- is caused by a virus infection
- your child's cough will be hoarse, sounding like a seal or a dog's bark
- an attack of croup can come on suddenly and be very frightening
- if your child's lips are blue or if breathing is very difficult, take him to casualty
- if the attack is not too severe, call the GP, then calm your child down and sit in the bathroom with the hot taps running and the door shut as the steam will ease breathing

Ear infections

- are especially common in the under fives and often follow a cold
- middle ear infections can be very painful and need prompt treatment as otherwise they may cause permanent hearing loss
- repeated ear infections need investigation by a specialist in order to prevent glue ear

YOU THE EXPERT

'When my baby had a cold, the health visitor showed me how to tickle her nostrils with some cotton wool. It made her sneeze, and of course that cleared her nose.' Ann Payne, St Albans

Hormone replacement therapy can relieve both the

HELP! MY TODDLER WON'T SLEEP

Parents accept that when their babies are tiny, they are likely to cry in the night. What no one tells parents is that their children's sleeping habits are likely to get worse as they grow older, not better. And of course, they can get out of bed too.

The main sleeping problems are

- won't go to bed
- gets up or screams in the middle of the night
- gets into your bed every night

If your child is still a babe, here's how to prevent these happening

- establish a bedtime routine, e.g. bath, story, bed
- don't rock him to sleep in your arms, but put him in his cot whilst dozy but still awake
- if your baby wakes in the night but doesn't cry loudly, let him settle himself
- if your baby wakes, be firm – avoid eye contact, don't play with him or give him drinks (other than water)

If you've already got a night-time horror, here are some tricks of the trade

- if he wakes and cries, let her cry for 5–10 minutes (no longer as by that time hysteria sets in)
- pick him up, cuddle him (but no more), wait till his crying subsides and then put him firmly back in the cot again

- gradually increase the initial crying time by a few minutes each time he wakes

This method only works if you are dedicated to breaking your child's bad sleeping habits. The first night will be awful, but providing you stick to your guns, it usually works within a few days. Try it over a holiday period or weekend. Other sleep problems are:

He won't go to bed at night

- have a bedtime routine. If he won't normally settle till 10 pm, it won't work if you first try it at 6 pm. Try it at 9.30 pm and then keep bringing it forward
- don't overstimulate him in the evening
- when you put him down, be firm and decisive about it and then beat a retreat

He comes into your bed at night

- the moment she appears, put him back firmly
- if he comes back, issue a stern warning and get your partner to return him
- don't lose your temper

The most important thing is to be firm and for both parents to be consistent. Once one weakens, you're sunk.

These ideas come from the splendid Dr Christopher Green whose book *Toddler taming* should be on every despairing parent's bookshelf.

physical and psychological effects of the menopause.

ASTHMA

In the UK, at least one child in seven has asthma and the number of children being diagnosed with the condition is increasing all the time. No one is quite sure why there should have been such a rapid rise in cases. Pollution is often blamed – but there's no scientific evidence this is the case, and anyway it's not the whole story because asthma is increasing all over the country, not just in the areas of greatest pollution.

How to recognise asthma in your child

- repeated attacks of wheezing or coughing, usually with colds

- a cough that keeps coming back or which is persistent, dry and irritating

- a cough that is often worse at night

- wheezing or coughing after exercise or excitement

- recurrent chest infections

In older children and adults, asthma can be diagnosed with a peak flow meter, but this is not effective in children under the age of six.

What triggers attacks? Attacks can be triggered by allergy, for instance to the house dust mite, pets, pollen, etc. but also by exercise, cigarette smoke, emotion or sudden exposure to cold air. Children's asthma is triggered in particular by colds and viruses (especially in the under fives).

Treatment There are two types of medicine – relievers and preventers. Relievers – such as Ventolin and Bricanyl are taken during attacks. If your child needs to use a reliever more than once a day, he or she might need preventer treatment. The most usual preventers are inhaled steroids (e.g. Becotide, Pulmicort). It is vital that these are taken regularly whether your child has an asthma attack that day or not. They may take 10–14 days to become fully effective.

Most people think that it's better not to take drugs if at all possible and think their asthmatic child would be better off without them, especially steroids. But these are completely different from the steroids sometimes used by bodybuilders and are given in tiny doses. Also because they are inhaled directly into the lungs, very little of the medicine gets into the bloodstream, so it carries a very small risk of side-effects.

There are over 30 different types of inhaler devices and your GP or asthma clinic nurse will help you to find the one that best suits your child. Under fives will usually need a spacer (a clear plastic inhaler add-on that makes it easier to use).

Play detective The best drug treatment is the one that uses the minimum of medication to achieve the desired effect. But if you can find the triggers of your child's asthma and avoid them, you may be able to reduce their medication.

Each year 110 000 people die from

What to do if your child has an asthma attack

- give your child the reliever treatment immediately – wait 5–10 minutes, and repeat until breathing is improved or help has arrived – reliever medication is safe so there is little danger of your child overdosing

- hold or sit the child in an upright position to assist breathing

- if the child does not significantly improve after reliever treatment or gets worse, call your doctor or ambulance (whichever is likely to be quicker) or take your child to hospital

Asthma management You will be able to work out a management plan for your child with the practice nurse or GP which will tell you

- what drugs to take when, at what dosage

- what signs and symptoms of worsening asthma to look out for

- when to increase or decrease the dose of regular medication

- when to call the doctor

Some children with asthma are encouraged to measure their lung function using a peak flow meter and adjust their asthma therapy accordingly. This is just as important for an asthmatic as it is for a diabetic to measure blood sugar daily.

Asthma at school In every class of 30 children, there will probably be at least four or five children with asthma – three of which are diagnosed, and two undiagnosed.

You need to talk to your child's teachers and explain the situation. The National Asthma Campaign has produced a School Asthma Card which doctors can complete with your child's details.

Some schools insist that inhalers are kept in the school office to be given out on request but this may prevent children having medicine when they need it most. Usually children are sensible enough to keep their inhaler with them. But they may need to be reminded to:

- take a dose of preventer medicine at lunchtime (if they need this four times daily)

- to use a relief inhaler before going out into the cold air, or before sport

YOU THE EXPERT

'My son was always losing his reliever, so I got him a special 'bumbag' to wear to school to keep it in.'
Stephanie James. Dalston

> **TOP TIP**
>
> Make sure *anyone* caring for your child knows about their asthma. Give them written information.

moking-related diseases in the UK.

It's only natural for new parents to worry about their baby and you may feel anxious about contacting the doctor because you're not sure whether your baby is really ill. Trust your instincts and whenever in doubt, ring your doctor.

Most GPs are very supportive of new parents and will arrange to see your baby at short notice without an appointment. You should always contact your doctor urgently whatever the time of day or night if your baby has any of the following symptoms.

- a fit (convulsion) or if the baby turns blue, is very pale or seems floppy
- has a very high temperature (over 39°C) especially if there's a rash (Calpol in the correct dosage is good for reducing temperature)
- difficulty breathing, breathing fast or grunting breathing
- unusually drowsy, hard to wake or doesn't seem to know you
- a temperature but the hands and feet are clammy

Other symptoms which can be serious and which should prompt a visit to the doctor are

- a hoarse cough with noisy breathing
- crying for an unusually long time, or in an unusual way or seeming to be in pain
- refusing feeds
- diarrhoea or vomiting, especially both together

Baby medicine tips You need to ask all the same questions about medicines for babies as the ones for adults given on p.3. Medicines used to be ready diluted for babies but are now dispensed with instructions on how to measure the correct dose for the age of your child. Ask for a liquid medicine measure (which looks like a syringe) from the pharmacist – it's more accurate than a teaspoon and less likely to spill. Ask for sugar free medicines – your baby's emerging teeth are very vulnerable. Don't ever give adult medicines to a baby and avoid using aspirin in babies and young children.

Immunisation Because immunisation has been so successful it's easy to forget how widespread, and how devastating, diseases like polio once were. Immunisation protects both individuals and whole communities from infectious diseases. The most usual vaccination programme is:

- DTP (diptheria, tetanus and pertussis (whooping cough) at 2, 3 and 4 months
- Polio – given by mouth at 2, 3 and 4 months plus booster doses later in childhood
- MMR – measles, mumps and rubella, given once, usually at 13 months
- Hib – protects against the bacteria that cause one form of meningitis, given at 2, 3 and 4 months

Alcohol is involved in about

Your teenagers may go through their adolescence with never a visit to the GP but there are some particular health problems that they face.

Painful periods In the first couple of years after your daughter starts her periods, they may be relatively pain free. But many teenagers will develop painful periods, which may be severe enough to make them vomit and certainly prevent them from going to school. One in three teenage girls report time off school because of periods. You may think that there is something very wrong, but this is unlikely to be the case and period pain does usually improve with age. Whatever you do, don't underestimate period pain in teenagers.

How to help
- choose painkillers wisely – those that contain anti-inflammatory agents such as Nurofen are the most effective
- a hot water bottle or hot bath can ease pain
- slow stretching exercises during the worst time and increased exercise in general will help
- if these measures are not enough, seek help from your GP

Your GP may prescribe stronger painkillers or suggest that your daughter goes on the pill. Period pain only occurs in menstrual cycles in which an egg is released. Being on the pill means that no egg is released during the cycle, and periods tend to be far less painful as a result. You may feel very unhappy about this, fearing that it will encourage earlier sexual activity. This is unlikely to be the case but discuss these issues with your daughter. Trust your daughter and realise that solving the misery of her period problems has to be your first concern.

Not eating properly One in three teenage girls are iron deficient, and the majority do not take in enough calcium for their daily needs. The reason for this may simply be that they are not eating enough food, or food of the right sort – probably because they are dieting. In addition, your teenager (with or without your knowledge) may be smoking.

This is a potent mix – although teenagers are resilient and may believe themselves to be healthy, the combination of dieting, lack of exercise and smoking could put them at considerable risk of a much earlier onset of osteoporosis, the brittle bone disease normally associated with the elderly. All you can do is try and ensure that your teenager has proper meals at home using foods in the proportions shown in The Balance of Good Health on page 16, and try and educate her about the dangers of not eating properly. A vitamin supplement may be the best solution, particularly if your child is a vegetarian who is eating a restricted range of foods (the best source of iron is meat).

Not eating enough It is generally accepted that young people, especially women, are preoccupied with their weight – 50 per cent of young females identify themselves as fat and 30 per cent have dieted at some time. Taken to extremes dieting can lead to anorexia nervosa.

Recognising anorexia Signs to look for are

- extreme food avoidance
- extreme physical activity
- avoidance of meal times
- obsession with daily weighing

But these have to be seen against a background of a personality whereby the child

- sets themselves very high standards
- is over complaint
- is a perfectionist
- is excessively orderly and tidy

If your child is underweight and exhibits several of these characteristics from **both** these lists, they may well be suffering from anorexia and you should seek help from your GP.

The Balance of Good Health

Fruit and vegetables

Bread, other cereals and potatoes

Puffed Wheat

HIGH FIBRE *Breakfast* FLAKES

PEAS

SWEETCORN

PEACH SLICES

MACARONI

LEMONADE

SEMI SKIMMED MILK

NUTS

BEANS

TUNA

CRISPS

LOW FAT NATURAL YOGURT

SPREADING FAT

Meat, fish and alternatives

Foods containing fat
Foods containing sugar

Milk and dairy foods

Physical activity is one of the best ways to relieve stress.

DRUG TAKING IN TEENAGERS

You need to set an example in the way that you yourself use alcohol, tobacco and medicines. Make sure, without being aggressive, that your views and feelings are known and you want your child to respect them.

All children can be tempted to take drugs – no matter what school they're at, no matter where they come from or how 'well brought up' they are. They take drugs for many reasons:

- curiosity
- pressure from friends because it's the 'in' thing boredom
- because they get a buzz from doing something their parents won't like and is illegal
- to escape from problems at home or at school

It's better that you talk to your child about drugs and what they might do if they are offered them, rather than ignore it and hope it won't happen. If you feel you don't know much about drugs, get *A parents' guide to drugs and solvents* from the HEA.

There are a number of signs which might suggest drug taking – but you need to be sure of your facts before you make any accusations.

- sudden changes of mood
- unusual irritability or aggression or bouts of sleepiness, or drowsiness
- unexplained loss of money or articles
- increased telling of lies or furtive behaviour
- unusual smells or stains on their bodies or around the home

If you have always thought you had a close relationship with your child, you may feel betrayed and hurt by the discovery that they are taking drugs. You shouldn't blame yourself, often drug taking is a passing phase and it's no reflection on what your child feels for you. It's tempting to go ballistic – but don't go over the top. It doesn't help. Be firm, consistent and caring – but disapproving and not just because drugs are illegal. Don't lecture, preach or bully your child.

- explain the reasons for rejecting drugs, including their illegality and health risks
- show that you will continue to support your child
- remember they may need more help than you can provide and be prepared to seek help from professional sources for both them and yourself
- be realistic about stopping, it's more likely to be gradual than immediate

Immunisation is the safest way to protect your child.

Teenagers today face greater degrees of stress in their lives than their parents did when they were teenagers. If you're the parent of a teenager, you may wonder how that can be – after all your teenager probably has many more material advantages than you had at their age. Yet for all that, teenagers are desperately vulnerable to stress. It comes from all quarters.

- pressure to achieve and do well at school conflicting messages from peers and parents about how to behave
- pressure to develop relationships and 'do it'
- pressures to smoke, drink or take drugs from peers and pressures not to from parents
- pressure from the media to be gorgeous, i.e. thin
- bullying from their peers if they do not conform to the norm in some way

All the tips on p.19 for dealing with stress apply to teenagers too. Although you may have a very good relationship with your children, don't be surprised or too hurt if there are things that they don't want to tell you.

- try not to be judgmental when your children make mistakes, because that's how they learn
- remember that they may not have the experience or knowledge to view problems in the same way as you do
- know how to access sources of professional support for your teenagers
- recognise when they are under strain and offer to listen
- realise how important their friends are to them
- take your children seriously
- value their opinions

Exams Of course exams are stressful, but today's teenagers may be under greater stress than you realise during exams. Parents have always told their children that good exam results may be their only passport to success in the future but the insecurity of today's employment patterns constantly serves to reinforce this.

Nag your teenagers to work hard by all means but as exams come up, ease off and be as supportive as you can. Here's a golden guide to beating exam stress.

- make a revision timetable so you feel more in control
- build flexibility into the timetable and don't set yourself unrealistic goals
- allow time off to relax, indulge in physical activity and have fun
- eat regular balanced meals and get plenty of sleep
- relax with a hot bath, warm drink and gentle music
- if you can't sleep, get up, make a drink and read something light

YOU THE EXPERT

'My brain went soggy if I stayed in all day revising, so I went out and played football in the afternoon. My mum went mad but I did alright, so it must have been good for me!' Peter Robinson, London

Nearly 50 per cent of men and 40 per

STRESS

Tension headaches, nervous diarrhoea, increased susceptibility to infection – all can be reactions to stress. In fact, some GPs think that stress-related illness accounts for about a tenth of all illness they see.

Life isn't as hard now as it was for people who lived through the '30s and '40s, but we face stresses of a different sort – uncertain employment, higher pressure to achieve and so on. And we no longer have the support in terms of extended families or close knit communities to deal with such pressures.

We would like to think that stress is caused entirely by external factors – changes in relationships, problems at work, financial difficulties at home and so on. Most stress, however, is self-generated because even though the external factor is the stimulus, it's how you react to it that is important. The pressures you create might include

- forcing yourself to work long hours
- lack of time for relaxation
- allowing yourself to become physically unfit
- having a negative self-image
- being uncertain about your goals in life
- believing that admitting to a problem is a sign of weakness
- keeping things bottled up inside

How to cope
The first step is to recognise that you need to do something about stress and to put aside some time for yourself.

1. Relax
Complementary therapies, particularly aromatherapy, massage and reflexology can help overcome stress – experiment with a few and see which one you find most relaxing. You may need to be taught how to relax – there are many self-help books and local classes that do this. It may seem like a contradiction, but physical activity is wonderfully relaxing and it's an essential part of stress management – start with gentle walking or swimming. Think about what you're eating and drinking too as this may be contributing to your problem – give yourself time to eat proper meals and keep your alcohol and caffeine intake to a minimum. And if you think smoking is relaxing, stop deluding yourself – it increases your heart beat and your blood pressure.

2. Work out how to change your life for the better
You may need help to do this, perhaps from a counsellor.

- be positive – change those things that can be altered, accept those that can't
- say 'no' more often – it will prevent you from getting overloaded
- don't compare yourself unfavourably with others
- set realistic goals and deal with your problems in small steps
- expect to make mistakes sometimes

YOU THE EXPERT

'Saying 'no' was a revelation. People respected me for saying it, but best of all, they stopped dumping all their jobs on me.' Rita Shamia Middlesborough

BREAST LUMPS

When a woman feels a lump in her breast, the first reaction is always panic and 'it must be cancer'. For nine out of ten women, it is not breast cancer.

In fact there are many causes of breast lumps, which vary with your age.

Fibro-adenomas These often develop in a woman's twenties, and are small lumps which move under the pressure of your finger (hence their other name of 'breast mice'). Doctors always used to be taught to remove all breast lumps, but it's now standard practice to leave benign small lumps such as these where they are.

If you are over 30 and have a single lump, it may be removed for analysis.

Breast cysts Tend to develop between the late 30s to 50s. They are smooth lumps containing fluid which can be withdrawn (aspirated) using a fine needle. They tend to recur.

Lumpy breasts Occurring at any age, lumpiness is felt all over the breasts, with several persistent lumps and is related to your menstrual cycle. Tell your GP about it, but generally he will be able to reassure you that this is just a normal part of breast development. It is not related to breast cancer.

Breast pain About 70 per cent of women will experience breast pain (mastalgia). For 40 per cent of these, the breast pain will be cylical (related to their periods), with the breasts feeling 'heavy' and tender to touch. Its cause is probably related to hormones and has been proved not to be related to water retention or stress.

- cut down saturated fats in your diet
- wear a well fitting bra
- see if cutting your caffeine intake will help
- if you are on the pill or using HRT, your problem may go if you come off them or change the type you are using
- try evening primrose oil for at least three months

If breast pain persists, your GP may prescribe a stronger medical grade of primrose oil or other drugs. Vitamin B6, diuretics and antibiotics have been shown not to work.

In women whose breast pain is not related to their cycle, the pain is usually muscular in origin and painkillers may help.

It isn't true that breast cancer is always painless but breast pain is only very rarely a symptom of cancer and almost never if it's associated with your cycle.

BREAST CANCER

What you can do to help yourself.

Be breast aware Knowing what's normal for you means that you notice any changes quickly.

- are both breasts still the same size and shape?
- is there any discharge from the nipples or swelling around them?
- is there any puckering or dimpling of the skin?
- is there a lump either in your breast or armpit?

What if I do find something? Tell someone quickly. Nine out of ten lumps will prove to be harmless. And if it were to be cancer, the earlier you have medical attention, the better.

Breast cancer is uncommon in young women

I'm 42 – why don't women of my age have mammograms every year? Under the age of 50, breast tissue is denser making it difficult for doctors to interpret X-rays correctly. Many women of this age might be told they had cancer, when in fact they didn't. Others might be falsely reassured. And in any case X-ray exposure should be kept to a minimum. If you are very concerned about this, or are at high risk, e.g. have a family history of breast cancer, your GP may refer you to a breast clinic for further advice and assessment.

I'm 65, what about me? Screening every 3 years is offered to all women aged 50–64. But if you're older you can also ask to be screened. It's a very sensible thing to do – and it's your right, so don't be afraid to ask.

My mother died of breast cancer, will it happen to me? Cancer is much more common as we get older. If your mother or other relative was over 65, her breast cancer is likely to be age related. If your mother or other close relative developed it before menopause, it's more likely that there is an inherited element – but it still doesn't necessarily mean you will get it. Talk to your GP about your fears and concerns.

I've heard about a test for breast cancer One in 20 women have an inherited form of breast cancer. Most of these women are from 'cancer families', where many relatives are affected by breast, ovarian or other cancers. The test, for the presence of the BRCA1 gene, which causes some of these inherited types of breast cancer, is available in the USA. However, there is concern about how the results should be interpreted. Also, a negative result doesn't mean you won't get breast cancer – just that your risk is lower than originally thought.

The earlier a breast cancer is diagnosed, the greater the chances of successful treatment. Five year survival rates are 84 per cent when the disease is detected at the earliest stage.

back pain as a cause of lost working days.

BACK PAIN

Back pain is one of the top ten reasons for people to consult their GPs and affects nearly three-quarters of us at some time during our lives.

When back pain strikes

- take a good painkiller, preferably one containing an anti-inflammatory such as ibuprofen, e.g. Nurofen

- rest for up to 48 hours

- about four times a day, try a hot and cold regime on the sore area – one minute of ice (using an ice pack or pack of frozen peas) followed by three minutes of heat using a hot water bottle or hot flannel. Repeat once.

- if pain isn't relieved after 48 hours, gets worse, or travels down your legs, see your GP

If the pain is relieved, you should return to your normal daily life – but take this opportunity to assess your lifestyle and find out what you have been doing to cause or aggravate your back problem. Could it be:

- sitting for long periods without support

- driving in hunched or cramped positions for a long time

- lifting objects which are too heavy or lifting them incorrectly

- using an awkward twisting movement

- sleeping on an old soft or sagging mattress

- being generally unfit (fit muscles are better able to withstand strain)

Physical activity is now recognised to be an important element in recovery from both acute back ache and chronic back pain. So, once your pain begins to ease off, you should think about some gentle exercises to improve your back's flexibility and strength. Sources of exercise plans are at the back of this booklet. If any exercise increases your back pain, you should stop. If you want to increase your fitness as well, good forms of exercise for back pain sufferers include:

- swimming – but not breaststroke as this puts strain on the spine

- cycling, preferably on a cycle without drop handlebars

If you have leg pain (sciatica) you may need to rest for longer than 48 hours.

Many types of back pain can be helped by manipulative techniques such as osteopathy, chiropractic or physiotherapy and your GP will usually be able to recommend someone. If not, you can find someone local through the representative bodies (addresses on p.48)

There are many different causes of back pain – so even if you think your pain is similar to a friend's, always check with your GP.

The good news is that 75 per cent of people suffering back pain recover within a month and 90 per cent within three months.

YOU THE EXPERT

'I always got backache after driving until a physiotherapist told me to put a rolled up towel in the hollow of my back when driving. It's really helped.' Fiona Hunter, Liverpool

TOP TIPS

- get up and stretch every 15 minutes when working over a desk

- don't carry one heavy shopping bag, distribute the weight better in two

- don't carry your baby on one hip

A peptic ulcer develops in about

SNORING

People laugh about snoring but it's no laughing matter. About 30 per cent of the adult population snores regularly. And men do it more than women – 50 per cent of middle-aged men snore, compared to only 14 per cent of middle-aged women.

Snoring can be very loud – the world's champion snorer produced 87.4 decibels – the same as a revving motorbike. Basically it occurs because the airways are narrowed or partially blocked, causing vibrations in the upper respiratory tract. Persistent snoring can wreck marriages.

Most people snore from time to time because:

- they've drunk too much alcohol
- they have hay fever, a cold or cough
- they are heavy smokers
- they are overweight

Whilst occasional snoring is normal, persistent snoring is not. It's a myth that snorers do it only on their backs – moderate to severe snorers snore in any position – and even when their mouths are closed. These snorers just can't help snoring.

Although heavy snorers seem to be sound asleep, snoring disturbs their sleep too and they may end up feeling permanently tired. Snoring combined with daytime exhaustion, irritability or changes in mood are symptoms of the condition called obstructive sleep apnoea. The sleeper actually stops breathing, briefly wakes and struggles to breathe again, often producing a mighty snore in the process. Partners often say that they think the sufferer has actually stopped breathing. It's important that the condition is recognised as it is associated with an increased rate of heart attack and stroke.

Usually sleep apnoea is diagnosed following an overnight stay in a sleep clinic. Many people with sleep apnoea are helped by wearing a special machine at night – it works like a vacuum cleaner in reverse and forces the airways to stay open. Surgery may also help some sufferers.

What you can do to help yourself.

- lose weight – excess fat around the throat narrows the airway
- stop smoking
- don't drink last thing at night
- sort out nasal congestion if this is a problem for you
- try one of the cheap patent anti-snoring devices which hold open the nostrils – most are available over the counter at your pharmacist
- contact the British Snoring and Sleep Apnoea Association for more information about the best type of anti-snoring device before parting with any money (see p.48)

YOU THE EXPERT

'My husband snored only when he lay on his back, so I sewed a cork to the back of his pyjamas - it stopped him lying on his back and his snoring wasn't half as bad.' Edith Mant, Cumbria

ne in eight people in the UK.

Half of all people whose bowel symptoms are investigated in hospital are diagnosed as having the Irritable Bowel Syndrome (IBS) and it is second only to back pain as a cause of lost working hours.

IBS affects the muscles of the bowel wall, making them work ineffectively. Sufferers may experience abdominal pain, constipation, diarrhoea or alternate bouts of both, together with other symptoms. The condition is also called spastic colon or mucous colitis. It affects all age groups but is twice as common in women as in men. It may start in early or middle age, despite previous good health. Although it's not life threatening, it is the source of great distress and much misery.

The causes are not fully understood but anything that depresses the body's defence system such as being physically run down after illness or which disturbs the natural balance of 'normal' bacteria in the gut, may be a trigger. Anxiety and tension don't cause the condition but tend to make it worse.

Sufferers are often worried that something is seriously wrong with them. But relief when their bowel is found to be 'normal', often turns to despair when their symptoms won't go away, despite nothing abnormal being identified.

Aromatherapy Relaxing oils include lavender, rose, clary sage, neroli and petitgrain. Remember essential oils must not be put directly on the skin. Use a carrier oil such as sweet almond if you are using them for massage.

TOP TIPS TO HELP YOURSELF

- drink more water, particularly on waking and between meals
- add more fibre – wholegrain bread, pasta and rice, fruit and vegetables – to your diet, although you should avoid bran as it makes things worse for some sufferers
- cut down on high fat foods
- take a bulk-forming agent which will stimulate gut movement, e.g. Isogel
- avoid laxatives
- stop smoking
- take more exercise
- practise relaxation techniques
- many sufferers find complementary medicines such as reflexology and aromatherapy especially helpful
- try to find out which foods trigger attacks and avoid them

YOU THE EXPERT

'*My IBS coincided with a very stressful time at work. Someone suggested exercise — so I started swimming three times a week, starting with just a few lengths. I find my symptoms are much more controllable now.*' Liz Weeks, Hunstanton

Walking briskly for thirty

There are two main types of peptic ulcer – gastric ulcers found in the stomach and duodenal ulcers found in the first part of the small bowel. Gastric ulcers are less common and are found in the older age group while duodenal ulcers are more common, occurring in all age groups but particularly in the 25–50s.

Some people with a peptic ulcer have no symptoms. Others have indigestion or a burning or gnawing pain in the abdomen, usually on an empty stomach, which may be relieved temporarily when they take indigestion remedies. Pain may also be felt in the back. Although the popular image of an ulcer sufferer is a stressed business man, forced to eat nothing but fish and milk puddings, this view is outdated.

TOP TIPS TO HELP YOURSELF

- stop smoking – the most important step
- avoid drinking coffee, tea and alcohol
- avoid using aspirin or other non steroidal anti-inflammatory drugs
- eat several small meals at regular intervals, rather than a few big ones

If indigestion symptoms persist, don't keep treating yourself – always tell your doctor as they may need to be investigated. Ulcers can be diagnosed by endoscopy (passing a viewing tube into the stomach) and need to be treated as otherwise there is a danger they may bleed or perforate the stomach wall.

Although antacids may help, your GP will probably prescribe acid reducing drugs. The best known are Zantac (ranitidine) and Tagamet (cimetidine). These effectively reduce acid secretions, so allowing your ulcer to heal – usually within to 6–8 weeks. But about 80 per cent of people find that their ulcer symptoms return again. If they do, your GP may suggest testing you for the presence of *Helicobacter pylori* (*H. pylori*).

H. pylori is a common bacteria found in the stomachs of at least 50 per cent of adults. Most get no symptoms, some get indigestion but only a few go on to get ulcers. It's thought that although *H. pylori* increases the production of stomach acid, it's the addition of lifestyle factors (such as smoking, diet etc) that cause ulcers to form.

One test to detect *H. pylori* is a breath test. This test is simple – swallow some special liquid and then breathe into a container. If the bacteria is detected, a two-week course of combined antibiotic and acid reducing drugs will usually eradicate the infection. Around 95 per cent of ulcers will be completely cured.

Stomach ulcers can also be caused, especially in the elderly, by a number of medicines of a type called non steroidal anti-inflammatory drugs (NSAIDS). These should be stopped.

| 25

TOP TIP

Don't go on treating indigestion symptoms with over the counter remedies if they persist – see your doctor

Problem periods are experienced by almost all women at some time in their lives and are one of the most common reasons for a woman to consult her GP. Too painful, too infrequent, too heavy, too short, too long, too often – in fact, literally just too bloody awful for many women!

Most periods start at around the age of 12–13 and finish in a woman's early fifties at the menopause. Most women will experience around 400 periods during their lifetime.

It's normal for periods to change with your age – for instance, cramps are more common in teenagers and young women, periods may get heavier in the mid thirties and infrequent approaching the menopause. They may not return for some months after a birth. It's normal too for some periods to be heavier or more painful than others. Only you know what's normal – and what's not – for you.

Contraception can make your periods
- lighter (the pill)
- more infrequent (the mini-pill and injectable contraceptives)
- heavier (the coil – IUD)

So when should you go to the doctor?
- if your periods have altered for three months or more and are causing you concern
- if your period pain or heavy blood loss is preventing you from doing things you would normally do – like going to work or shopping
- if your periods are very infrequent or irregular

You should always tell your doctor if
- you are bleeding after making love
- if you suddenly start bleeding after the menopause
- if you are bleeding between periods

Women were often too embarrassed to seek help for periods and thought they should just put up with them. Doctors deal with period problems all the time and will be glad to see you and to help you.

Cycle length varies from an average of 35 days at age 12, to a minimum of 27 at 43 to 52 days at age 55. Only 12 per cent of women have the 'normal' 28 day cycle.

Very few or no periods If your periods have always been very irregular, it is possible that you have an underlying gynaecological condition. It is important that you see your GP and he may refer you to someone for specialist help, particularly if you want to get pregnant.

If you had normal periods and are now having very few, it could be:

- because of a sudden change in weight
- because you have been dieting or have anorexia
- you are an athlete or ballet dancer and have been training very hard lately
- because of stress caused by recent exams, bereavement or illness

Death rates from coronary heart disease in

You might like not having periods but six months or more without them means that, even if you are young, you are at risk of osteoporosis and need help. Hormonal treatment or sometimes just time and putting on (or losing) a bit of weight may be the answer.

Painful periods Some women always have painful periods (dysmenorrhoea), others only in their teens (see p.15). If your periods suddenly become painful, talk to your GP as you may have developed a pelvic infection, which needs urgent treatment, or possibly a condition called endometriosis.

The lining of your womb contains a cocktail of hormone – like substances called prostaglandins. When the normal balance of these is disturbed you may suddenly get a much more painful period, with cramps and pain in your thighs and back. Medicines like aspirin and ibuprofen (Nurofen) work against prostaglandins, which is why they can be effective for painful periods.

If you always have period pain and have something important like an exam or interview – or even your wedding – on the same day as your period, ask your GP. He can give you a hormone treatment to delay your period.

Heavy periods Average blood loss is about 35 ml (a cupful) but a few women can lose up to as much as 1000 ml a month. A heavy period is defined as losing more than 80 ml of blood.

Heavy periods can be caused by

- fibroids and polyps (non-cancerous growths in the womb)
- gynaecological conditions such as endometriosis pelvic infection
- the approach of the menopause, although generally periods get lighter and more irregular

But in over 50 per cent of cases, no cause can be found. Heavy periods may make you feel very tired and cause you embarrassment and inconvience. You don't have to put up with them. Assuming there's no identifiable cause, what can be done?

- the contraceptive pill will lighten your periods (you can carry on taking the pill if you are over 35, provided that you are a non-smoker)
- there are a range of medicines, some of which reduce blood loss by 60 per cent, which can be taken at the beginning of, or through, your period
- you can have the lining of your womb scraped (endometrial ablation/resection)
- if nothing else has worked, and periods are ruling your life, a hysterectomy may be suggested

Did you know? Menstrual blood doesn't clot (if it did it would soon gum up your womb). The clots you see if you have heavy periods are just balls of red blood cells.

'People think doctors have magic wands which they can wave which will make losing weight easy. Believe me, if I had a magic wand, I would have used it on myself long ago!' GP

We're gradually becoming a nation of fatties but where are you on this chart?

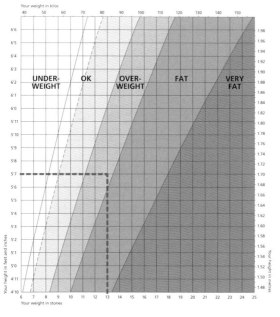

Measure across from your height to your weight to see which weight category you are in.

How to lose weight

Don't diet, change your diet

Nobody can sustain a crash diet for long, and the weight soon piles on again. Plan a healthier diet, with more vegetables and fruit and replace foods containing fat or sugar with starchy fibre-rich foods like bread, pasta and rice and you will find the weight comes off naturally – and for life (see p.16).

Exercise more

It's not something to do with your glands or having heavy bones. You take in more energy in the form of food than your body is able to use. Step up your exercise, and speed up the weight loss.

Do it with a friend

Sometimes it really helps to have some moral encouragement – so go for weight loss with a friend or join a club.

The loudest snore is

SMOKING

Most people who smoke say that they'd like to give up.

They've seen some of the facts about smoking.

- that smokers are at greater risk of illness and early death
- that 80 per cent of Britain's 30,000 annual lung cancer deaths are caused by it
- that 20 per cent of deaths from coronary heart disease are smoking related
- that 17,000 children are admitted to hospital each year because their parents smoke
- that each year smoking kills twenty times the number of people killed in car crashes in the UK

In fact, if you're a smoker, the single most positive thing you can do to improve your health is give up the fags.

How to do it Nobody ever said giving up was easy. If you want to stop, be clear about why you want to stop, prepare yourself to stop by writing up a list of all your reasons and decide a plan of action.

I need help

- ask your partner or friends to support you
- ring the Quitline on 0800 00 22 00 and get them to send you a Quitpack
- see if there is a stop smoking clinic at your GP's surgery

BUT

Surely it's too late to stop now – the damage is already done In fact some benefits start really quickly – you cough less and you breathe more easily after exercise. Within 10–15 years, your chances of lung cancer and heart attack aren't that much different from a non-smoker.

The withdrawal symptoms were awful last time Learn from them to make stopping easier this time. Symptoms such as hunger, disturbed sleep and irritation won't last long - no more than a month.

Won't I put on weight? You don't have to put on weight, and if you do, it'll only be a few pounds. Just try not to eat more when you stop.

So now you're ready

- choose a day and stick to it
- get rid of your cigarettes, lighters and ashtrays the day before
- make sure your help is in place, and you've told your friends, family and work colleagues
- make sure you reward yourself with little treats each day you succeed – you could even plan a holiday or buy a new outfit with the cash you save
- if you feel tempted, read your list of reasons to remind yourself why you are stopping

How long will it take?

It normally takes about 3 months before you will be able to think of yourself as a non-smoker. Most smokers are able to resist the occasional 'wouldn't it be nice to have one' feeling. Never risk 'just one cigarette'.

But one day you'll wake up and realise that you don't miss it any longer and then you've cracked it – you're a non-smoker. Congratulations!

TIPS TO SUCCEED

- if you smoke most when you're busy, choose a holiday period to give up
- if you smoke with a coffee or a drink, change your habits for a bit and drink juice instead of coffee
- plan in advance how you'll cope with difficult situations, like a party
- buy some sugar-free gum if you need to put something in your mouth
- drink juice or eat fruit – Vitamin C helps the body rid itself of nicotine

like a revving motorbike.

BLOOD PRESSURE

Blood pressure is a bit mysterious. You have it but you can't feel it and when there's something wrong with it, you may be the last one to know. Yet for all that, blood pressure is the key to your good health.

What exactly is it? Your heart has to force your blood through all your blood vessels – blood pressure is a measure of that force. If your blood vessels have become narrowed – for instance, by fatty deposits on their walls – more force is needed to push blood through them – and your blood pressure will rise.

Blood pressure changes minute by minute, depending on what you are doing. For instance, it rises during exercise but falls during sleep. Your blood pressure increases with your age.

What are they doing when they put that cuff thing on you? When your blood pressure is measured, two pressures are recorded. Systolic, the highest, is the pressure created as the heart muscle contracts and squirts blood out of the heart. Diastolic is the pressure recorded whilst the heart is relaxing between beats. Blood pressure is measured in millimetres of mercury (mmHg).

Because blood pressure is naturally so variable, hypertension (permanently raised blood pressure) is only confirmed when a person's blood pressure at rest is raised on three separate occasions.

Why is hypertension bad? Your heart has to work harder to maintain such a high blood pressure and your blood vessels aren't designed to withstand this force. So, there is an increased risk of stroke and also coronary heart disease. Very high blood pressure can also affect kidneys and sight, but very few people will ever have noticeable symptoms of their hypertension.

So, it's a silent killer Neither you nor your doctor can tell whether your blood pressure is likely to be raised without measuring it. If you don't know it's high, you can't prevent its potentially devastating effects.

And dead common Hypertension is one of the most common reasons why people visit their GPs. About 1 in 5 of the adult population have it, although 90 per cent will have no obvious cause for their raised blood pressure.

So how do I avoid it?
- give up smoking
- reduce your fat intake
- lose weight if you are overweight
- get out and do some exercise
- cut back your alcohol consumption
- reduce your salt intake
- learn how to relax and manage stress

Doing the things above may be enough not only to prevent hypertension but to reduce it if it has been diagnosed. If not, your doctor may have to prescribe anti-hypertensive drugs to help.

YOU THE EXPERT

'I have low blood pressure and often feel faint if I get up suddenly. So, I have a hand grip and squeeze it hard just before I get up – doing that makes your blood pressure rise momentarily and stops you feeling wobbly. Simple.' Mr C Owens, Herts

A healthy lifestyle can reduce the risks of heart disease associated with a week or more, and eat healthily – plenty of fruit and vegetables, bread,

It never occurs to many women that they might be at risk of heart disease. In fact, most women think of heart attacks as something that only happens to men. 'When I had chest pain it never crossed my mind that it might be my heart' is a typical woman's comment.

Actually coronary heart disease is the largest single killer of women, claiming more lives than lung cancer and all the female cancers together. Whilst it is true that in the 35–44 age group coronary artery disease kills six times as many men as women, in the 55–70 age group, the death rates are pretty much equal.

Before the menopause women are protected from heart disease by their hormone oestrogen. However, this protection isn't foolproof – 25 per cent of heart attack deaths in women are in those under 45. First heart attacks are more likely to be fatal in women than men but the slightly better news is that women are more likely to have some prior warning in the form of angina than a man.

So what should women look for?

- a tightening or pain in the chest brought on by exertion which is relieved by rest
- pain in the arm or neck, without chest pain, brought on by exertion and relieved by rest
- chest pain which comes on suddenly whilst they are resting or at night

Which women are more at risk?

- if you are overweight
- if you lead a sedentary lifestyle
- if you smoke
- if you have high blood pressure
- if you have high blood cholesterol
- if you are diabetic
- if you have reached the menopause

It's not just whether you are overweight that is important in determining your risk from heart disease. It's where you carry your fat. Women who carry most of their excess weight around their middles, as happens after the menopause, are more at risk.

Your waist/hip ratio is an important measure of your risk – to work this out, measure your waist and hips, then divide the waist measurement by the hip measurement. The answer should be under 0.8. If not, you should try losing weight, see p.28.

diabetes – don't smoke, be moderately active for 30 minutes on 5 days cereals and pasta, cut down on fat, sugar and salt, drink sensibly.

MENOPAUSE

The menopause is an important crossroads in their life for many women and if you view it positively, it can be very rewarding. It marks the end of one part of your life – but the beginning of a new one.

Most women will have their last period around the age of 50. The average age of menopause is 51.

About three-quarters of women will experience symptoms of the menopause such as hot flushes, problems sleeping, vaginal dryness, depression, etc., some many years before their last period. Only 1 in 3 women will find their symptoms so distressing that they seek help.

How do I know I've definitely reached the menopause? Rising blood levels of the hormone FSH signal the approach of the menopause. Above a certain level indicates that menopause has occurred. Your GP may be able to arrange an FSH blood test.

Alternatives to HRT

Not every menopausal woman will be prescribed HRT (see p.33) or choose to take it, although you are strongly advised to do so if you are at risk of osteoporosis or coronary heart disease (see p.33). Here are some alternatives

- exercise – this maximises your internal oestrogens produced when fat is broken down, as well as keeping your bones strong, reducing your risk of heart disease and maintaining your joint flexibility

- complementary therapies such as aromatherapy, homeopathy and acupuncture to overcome menopause symptoms

- diet – at the menopause, women need to reconsider their diets as their need for some minerals and vitamins increases, while their calorie requirements fall. Reduce your fat, sugar, salt and caffeine intake. Increase fruit and vegetables, dairy products and fluids. Take care with alcohol as it makes hot flushes worse.

- stop smoking – it speeds up bone loss and makes flushes and night sweats worse

YOU THE EXPERT

'I was very well and didn't want to take HRT, but I did suffer from vaginal dryness which made sex difficult. I was too embarrassed to talk to my GP but when I finally plucked up courage, he was really understanding with lots of ideas to help. So my advice is don't suffer in silence.' Anon, Bedford
And

'Hot flushes were a problem, so I always wore several layers of thin clothing. That way, I could always take something off!' Mrs D Usher, Enfield

HORMONE REPLACEMENT THERAPY

Hormone replacement therapy (HRT) provides the hormones the body lacks as a result of the menopause. Unlike the pill which adds hormones to the body, HRT restores hormones to their natural level.

HRT can be taken as a variety of pills, as an implant, as an adhesive skin patch or a gel.

Women used to be given oestrogen alone but this meant that the lining of the womb grew too thick, increasing the risk of cancer of the womb. HRT is safer now because another hormone called progestogen is added but this has the disadvantage of causing a monthly bleed similar to a period. This is the main side-effect of HRT. However, there are now some 'no bleed' types – the synthetic hormone Livial and also continuous combined HRT (e.g. Kliofem, Premique). Another new development is long cycle HRT which allows a bleed only every three months.

Other side-effects include fluid retention (slight weight gain and perhaps ankle swelling), nausea and breast tenderness. Don't be put off by these side-effects – most only last a couple of months. If you feel no better after 3 months, ask your GP to either adjust your dose of HRT or recommend a different type.

Relief from menopausal symptoms is immediate but if you want the long-term benefits of HRT, you need to take it for at least five years.

Who should take HRT?

- women who have had an early menopause (before 45) or who had their ovaries removed
- women who have had a hysterectomy as 25 per cent will become oestrogen deficient within 2 years, even though they have not reached their menopause
- women who are at risk of osteoporosis
- women with a history of heart disease

Who shouldn't take HRT?

- women who have had cancer of the breast or womb
- women who have had recent blood clots
- women with kidney or liver disease

High blood pressure is *not* a reason to avoid HRT but it needs to be sorted out before HRT is started.

Doesn't HRT cause breast cancer?

If you take HRT for a long time (more than 10 years) the risk of breast cancer is increased slightly. However, on the positive side, your risk of osteoporosis will be reduced by 50–75 per cent and your risks from coronary heart disease will also fall.

YOU THE EXPERT

'I was disappointed by HRT at first. But I persevered and tried several different types until I found one that really suited me.' S Lindsay, Wiltshire

– airway, breathing, circulation

OSTEOPOROSIS

Osteoporosis is a disease which makes bones so porous and brittle that they break very easily. A minor fall can then result in a facture, usually of the hip, spine or wrist.

Although some bone loss is normal with age for both men and women, it is women who are especially vulnerable. However, osteoporosis is not a disease just of the elderly – thousands of women in their 50s have it and suffer painful fractures as a result.

A fracture might not sound very serious but 40 people die each day as a result of fractures due to osteoporosis. And more women die after hip fracture than from cancer of ovaries, cervix and womb combined. If the bones in the spine become weak because of osteoporosis, they crush together, resulting in back pain, loss of height and a curved spine.

Osteoporosis is a silent disease. Often a person only discovers that they have it when they suffer their first fracture. By this time, over a third of the skeleton may have been lost already.

What causes osteoporosis?
The skeleton is a living tissue – the body constantly removes old bone and puts new bone in its place. In women, the hormone oestrogen helps maintain bone density by slowing down the natural bone destruction process and improving the absorption of calcium from the diet. When the ovaries start to fail at menopause, and oestrogen levels fall, bone begins to be lost. A number of diseases are also associated with brittle bones.

Who is at risk?
- women who have had an early menopause (before the age of 45)
- women who have had a hysterectomy (especially if both ovaries have been removed)
- women who have missed periods for six months or more because of severe loss of weight, excessive exercise, etc
- men and women who have taken corticosteroid drugs for a long time
- men and women who are heavy smokers and drinkers
- men and women who have been immobile for long periods

There is some evidence that women who have close relatives with osteoporosis are more at risk.

How to prevent osteoporosis
Make sure that you build up strong bones before you reach 35 (the age when your bones are at their strongest and healthiest) by

- taking regular load bearing exercise such as walking
- making sure you have enough calcium in your diet
- not smoking
- not drinking too much

Calcium   As we age, our bodies begin to lose calcium and our ability to absorb it decreases. To use calcium effectively, the body also needs Vitamin D. At certain times of your life, such as adolescence, pregnancy and old age it is especially important to have a calcium rich diet. Calcium alone will not prevent osteoporosis, but it will help protect your skeleton for this serious disease.

A woman's need for calcium rises from 1000 mg a day between 20–45years of age, to 1500 mg a day when she is over 45.

The best sources of calcium are milk, cheese and yoghurt. If you are watching your weight, fat free varieties may contain as much calcium, if not more. Canned fish is a particularly good source. Although leafy vegetables such as spinach contain calcium, it is not in an easily absorbed form.

How is osteoporosis diagnosed?   The usual method is using a DXA scan. Normally, bones in the spine and one hip are scanned. It takes about 30 minutes and isn't unpleasant in any way. Although X-rays can be used to spot fractures, they're not much good for assessing bone density.

If you are at risk, take HRT   Although it's important to increase your intake of calcium, exercise more, etc. it's not the whole answer. Without oestrogen, your body won't be able to use calcium properly, no matter how much you take.

If you fall into any of the risk groups or if bone scans reveal a low bone density, HRT is essential. It will help prevent osteoporosis (the risk of fracture is reduced by 50 per cent for women taking it at menopause), it halts bone loss in sufferers and depending on the type of HRT, may also replace bone in some women, although sadly not repair damage that has already occurred.

What about other treatments? If you are unable or do not wish to take HRT, other treatments include etidronate (mainly for spinal problems), calcium supplements, etc., but none of these will prevent osteoporosis.

A TIP FOR HEALTHY BONES

Jump up and down for healthy bones – a new study has shown that a simple routine of 50 small jumps on the spot can help keep bones strong.

YOU THE EXPERT

'I found hanging the washing out really difficult. Now I leave an old chair in the garden and put the washing basket on – it stops all that bending and stretching.' Audrey Cornish, Stafford

periods during their lifetime.

DIABETES

Around 3 per cent of the population in the UK have diabetes – that's well over a million people. But a further million people in the UK may have diabetes without knowing it.

What are the symptoms of undiagnosed diabetes?

- having a dry mouth and being thirsty all the time
- passing large amounts of urine
- being very tired
- losing weight
- have blurred vision
- having itchy genitals

There are two types of diabetes. Insulin dependent diabetes (Type 1) is the more severe and usually first appears before the age of 40. Insulin is a hormone produced in the pancreas which helps glucose (sugar) enter cells so it can be used as a fuel by the body. But in Type 1 diabetes most or all of the cells producing insulin in the pancreas have been destroyed. It is treated with injections of insulin and by diet.

Non-insulin dependent diabetes (Type 2) develops in people over the age of 40. It is most common amongst the elderly and overweight. Although the body is still producing insulin, it cannot produce enough for its needs or the insulin it does make is not being used properly. It is treated by diet alone or by diet and tablets or sometimes by diet and insulin injections.

The tendency to develop this second type of diabetes is passed from one generation to the next although the development of the condition is not automatic.

I've only got mild diabetes Even though you may be able to control your diabetes by diet alone, there's no such thing as mild diabetes. Everyone who has diabetes is at risk of developing complications, so it's very important that you follow a healthy lifestyle and maintain a good control of your blood glucose by having regular checks with your doctor.

What are the complications of diabetes? People with diabetes have an increased risk of heart disease and stroke. The combination of diabetes and other factors such as being overweight, having high blood pressure, high fat levels, smoking and taking little exercise all increase your risk. But you can do a great deal to reduce your risk.

- regular exercise will help you lose weight and reduce your blood pressure
- changes in the way you eat will help your weight and reduce your fat levels
- stopping smoking will make a real difference to your health

Controlling your diabetes also reduces the risk of other possible long-term complications of diabetes including eye, feet and kidney problems.

Now I know I'm diabetic, will I need to eat special foods? You don't need special diabetic foods. And you don't have to cut out things like biscuits and cakes completely – you can still eat them occasionally as part of an overall healthy diet. But there are some special things that you do need to do.

- try and cut down on fat – avoid fried and fatty foods such as butter, margarine, cheese and fatty meats which can all make you gain weight. And don't forget the hidden fats in biscuits, cakes and crisps. Use reduced fat spreads and skimmed or semi-skimmed milk

- eat more high fibre foods, especially things like beans, peas, lentils and fruit as the fibre in these slows down the rate at which your body absorbs carbohydrate

- try to cut down your sugar intake including sugar, sweets and sugary drinks. Use artificial sweeteners, diet drinks, etc.

- plan your meals around starchy foods such as bread, potatoes, rice, pasta and cereals which will help keep your blood sugar in the normal range

- eat regular meals

- cut down on your salt intake

- if you drink alcohol do so in moderation (2–3 units a day for women, 3–4 for men). And never drink alcohol on an empty stomach

As an example of what can be achieved, one insulin dependent diabetic woman gave up her job when she was diagnosed and trained to be a nurse. She specialised as a diabetic nurse and worked on the same ward in Alnwick where she herself was admitted. Now retired she remains very fit and regularly cycles 50 miles with her husband on a tandem.

Regular check-ups One of the most important things you can do to help yourself if you are diabetic is to ensure that you go to your GP or diabetic clinic for regular check-ups.

YOU THE EXPERT

'I was never very good at exercising but when I was diagnosed I got a dog – now I have to walk every day.' Ann Walker, Middlesborough

'Never walk around the house with bare feet – your feet can become less sensitive when you have diabetes, and if you stand on something sharp, the wound will take a long time to heal.' Millie McNab, Fulham

TOP TIPS

- find out as much as you can about the disease

- get organised – managing diabetes is all about organisation

- remember, healthy eating is the key to diabetic control

- take a list of questions when you go to the diabetic clinic so you don't forget any

- join the British Diabetic Association, as guidelines about the disease can change

ARTHRITIS

Rheumatism or arthritis? Arthritis is a disease which attacks the joints, sometimes leaving them damaged. Rheumatism is a more general term covering aches and pains in the bones, muscles, joints or tissues surrounding the joints, so rheumatism includes arthritis. There are over 200 types of arthritis.

Rheumatoid arthritis This is the most severe form. It causes inflammation of the joint lining. This results in pain, makes you feel ill and damages the joint. It may affect many joints as well as other organs in the body, e.g. the lungs. Some forms are auto-immune in origin (the body's defence system attacks its own tissue). It requires specialist assessment and treatment.

Osteoarthritis Osteoarthritis is the more common type. It generally starts in middle age and most commonly troubles older people but it is not caused by your joints 'wearing out', although it may follow damage to a joint earlier in your life. It has been shown that people inheriting a particular gene are more likely to develop it but this isn't the whole story as there are probably many other factors involved too.

Osteoarthritis can be painful but it does not lead to rheumatoid arthritis and it won't spread to all your joints, but probably just affect one or two. The pain sometimes gets better with time. If a particular joint is very badly affected, modern medicine has lots to offer, in the form of over the counter painkillers or non-steroidal anti-flammatory drugs available on perscription. If these do not work, joint replacement is now a highly successful option.

Diet There is now evidence that cutting down on saturated fats – red meat, full fat milk, etc. – can reduce the inflammation in the joints of people who suffer from all forms of arthritis.

In addition, particular foods may trigger inflammation in sufferers – although these differ from person to person, so don't be disappointed if what works for a friend, doesn't work for you.

If you remove an item from your diet, only for your symptoms to get worse over the next three or four days before improving, it may be an indication of food allergy. If you are making major changes to your diet, consult a dietitian who will help you ensure that you are still getting all the nutrients you need.

Fasting for a short period may also improve symptoms but be careful as fasting is not good for your health in general and symptoms generally quickly return.

Consuming more essential fatty acids – the sort that are in fish oils and evening primrose oil – can also reduce inflammation but be wary about taking too much cod liver oil or halibut liver oil as both are toxic in excess.

Losing weight One of the most important reasons to reconsider your diet if you are arthritic, is if you are overweight. Your hip and knee joints carry at least four times your body weight, so it's not surprising that people who are too heavy suffer from osteoarthritis in their legs. But it's not simply that the joints can't bear the load, those who are overweight are also more likely to develop osteoarthritis in their fingers and hands too.

What can I do to help myself?

Anything that you can do to help yourself will make you feel more in control of your symptoms – and that in itself will make you feel better.

Drug treatments

Painkillers can help joint pain from arthritis, e.g. paracetamol, codeine.

However, some painkillers such as non steroidal anti-inflammatory drugs can also be effective and can either be bought from the pharmacist, or stronger ones obtained on prescription, e.g. diclofenac. Two or three different mild ones may work better than one strong one.

Although inflammation isn't typically a feature of osteoarthritis, anti-inflammatory drugs, such as ibuprofen are often prescribed and are very helpful, although these drugs may also cause indigestion and ulcers. They are often prescribed to take at night as this is the best way to ease morning stiffness. They can also be taken in the form of a gel to rub into the affected joint.

Other stronger drugs such as steroids or ones that damp down the immune system may be appropriate for more severe forms of arthritis such as rheumatoid.

Practical tips

If your joints are tender and swollen – heat may be the best solution. Try a hot water bottle (but be careful not to burn yourself), a good soak in a hot bath or a visit to a steam room or sauna.

YOU THE EXPERT

'When my knee joint is stiff, I rub in one of those warming rubs, wrap my knee around with clingfilm and then put a hot wet towel around that. It's really effective.' *Elise Miller, Preston*

Hip replacement is a remarkably successful operation that has transformed the lives of hundreds of people who suffered many years of severe pain and stiffness.

Before the operation

- try to keep as full a range of mobility as possible in the hip
- exercise to keep thigh muscles (the 'quads') strong and stretch the hip – swimming, cycling, resting lying face down are all good
- keep your weight down
- get fit for your operation
- cut out smoking

After the operation

- slowly increase your exercise to strengthen the hip
- maintain the range of mobility
- go for short walks regularly – you should be walking within a week and by the time you leave hospital, be walking up and down stairs with a stick
- don't walk with a limp, learn to use the correct walking pattern
- for the first 6–10 weeks
  - don't lie or roll onto the operated side
  - don't bend the hip beyond 90°
  - don't take the operated leg across your midline
  - don't twist or swivel the operated leg when turning
  - if your pain has eased dramatically, you may be tempted to try and rush around like a two-year-old. Don't!
- don't be afraid to bend your leg but take care not to bend it too far
- you should be able to garden, but beware of getting your leg into an awkward position
- exercise classes (providing your instructor knows you've had a replacement hip), ballroom dancing and cycling will soon all be possible

Keeping fit as you get older If you have had a replacement hip, or if you have arthritis you may think that exercise is not for you. If you have osteoarthritis you may think that exercise will damage your joints because you have heard that arthritis is caused by joint 'wear and tear'.

It is important to rest if your joints are particularly inflamed and swollen. But exercise helps keep your muscles strong and prevents your joints from becoming stiff and painful. If you let your muscles become weak, you will put more strain on your joints, and it will be harder for you to get around and make it more likely that you will fall and injure yourself. Remember, although moving may hurt, not moving destroys.

Arthritis sufferers will benefit from exercises for specific joints and problem areas as well as from general exercise.

You need

- to keep your joints moving
- to improve the strength of your muscles
- to increase your fitness and stamina

Designed for you Ask your doctor or physiotherapist for some exercises tailored to your particular needs. Some will help build muscle strength, some will be for joint mobility.

Muscle strength Strengthening the muscles protects the joints from abnormal pressure which might cause further damage.

If you have arthritis in your knees, it's especially important to strengthen the muscles on the front of your thighs (the quadriceps) as it will help prevent further knee

disability. Bowling is both general exercise, and an exercise for those quad muscles.

General fitness Walking and cycling are both good forms of exercise, which involve the whole body. Swimming is especially good because your entire weight is supported in the water.

- start gently and if you begin to hurt, stop
- it's better to do a little exercise often, than do a lot in one go
- as you find exercise easier, gradually increase the amount you do

YOU THE EXPERT

'I found it difficult to get in the car after my op. But if you sit in backwards, and then swing your legs in, it's much easier.' *Jack Baldwin, London*

working days are lost through back pain.

PROSTATE PROBLEMS

The prostate gland lies at the base of the man's bladder. It surrounds the urethra – the tube that leads from the bladder to the penis – and is normally about the size of a walnut. It's job is to add fluid to the sperm as they are ejaculated. There are three main prostate problems.

Prostatitis, an infection of the prostate affecting mainly younger men.

Prostate cancer, which is the second largest cause of cancer for men.

Enlarged prostate, (also called BPH) which is extremely common in older men.

Enlarged prostate – over the age of 50, one in three men will develop troublesome urinary symptoms because of this, including:

- difficulty in starting to urinate

- having a dribble rather than a steady flow of urine

- pain or a burning feeling on urinating

- finding you need to go again, even though you've only just been

- having to get up frequently in the middle of the night

What will my GP do?
He will want to examine you so that the size and feel of your prostate can be assessed. Your urine may be tested for infection and for sugars (urinary problems are also associated with diabetes). As a screening test for prostate cancer, he may take a sample of blood to measure the level of prostate specific antigen (PSA), although this test is not very accurate.

How can it be treated? With drugs. There are three main types of drug, including a new form of hormonal treatment which shrinks the prostate (although this is slow to work and suitable for mild to moderate cases only).

With surgery. Either part or all of your prostate can be removed or by inserting a device into the prostate which keeps it open.

How to help yourself
- see your doctor – don't just think 'it's just old age'

- don't be tempted to cut down your daily fluid intake – all it will do is concentrate your urine and make bladder infection more likely

- cut down your fluid intake at night

YOU THE EXPERT

'I didn't drink anything for about 3 hours before I went out to the cinema in the evening – it meant I didn't miss any of the film.' G Kingsland, Solihull

CARING FOR SOMEONE WHO IS CONFUSED

More and more people are living longer and therefore diseases which were once rare are now much more common. Dementia is the result of a disease in which the cells of the brain die more quickly than they should. It produces loss of memory, confusion, odd behaviour and personality changes. It affects 6 in 100 people over 65, but 1 in 5 people over 85. So very many of us will have older relatives who will be affected.

There are many reasons why people find themselves looking after someone at home who is confused. Mostly it is because you love them, sometimes it is out of duty, sometimes there is no choice. For many carers it is an unwelcome and frightening prospect.

You may have suspected for some time that something is wrong. You may have tried to find an explanation – 'she's been doing too much' or persuaded yourself that this is just what happens to people as they get older.

Once a diagnosis of dementia has been made, you may feel overwhelmed by the enormity of it all, and be very anxious about the future and how you will cope. Often carers feel angry that this has happened. You may want to carry on caring for someone at home as long as you can, but you will certainly need help. Don't wait until you're desperate before you ask.

Help for you the carer
- talk to your GP. Be firm and persistent if he is not immediately helpful, as he is the key to all the services provided by the NHS, including help at home
- make sure you get a complete break even if it's through day care just one day a week
- talk to other carers as they are the people who will understand your problems best
- share the responsibility with other members of the family, or with friends and neighbours

There are often many more organisations available to help than you realise. Some voluntary organisations may offer help with practical tasks in the home or a meals on wheels service. They can supply safety aids and sometimes a laundry service.

Getting financial help Caring may alter your financial circumstances considerably – you may have to give up work, find more money for fuel bills. Find more money for special aids. You may be entitled to cash and other help from Social Security. The Benefit Enquiry Line (0800 88 22 00) gives free confidential advice. It's open 9am-6.30pm, weekdays and from 9am-1pm on Saturdays.

Caring at home
- try and keep things normal as long as possible. Don't give up going to the pub, football or cinema together unless it stops being a pleasure
- retain the sufferer's independence as long as possible – the more they can do for themselves, the less work for you and the more dignity for them
- try to avoid confrontation. Arguments are fruitless and just make you angry and frustrated

as fat and 30 per cent have dieted at some time.

- avoid crises – sufferers may get very confused by sudden change, having to hurry or too many people, so try and avoid such situations
- make things simple – don't offer too many choices
- establish routines
- make things safer – fit extra stair rails, secure loose mats, etc.
- try to make sure the sufferer continues to eat properly and has daily exercise

When you find yourself unable to cope 'Putting someone in a home' is an emotive phrase which makes all of us feel guilty, let alone the carer. But there's no need for guilt at all. Instead, be positive about how well you've coped so far in the circumstances and recognise when the needs of the sufferer begin to put your own health at risk, particularly if you too are getting on in years.

Getting permanent care The availability of permanent care varies enormously across the country.

It's possible to arrange it yourself, or through social services and the sufferer's GP or specialist.

Your choice of private care depends on what you can afford although there is state help in some cases.

You may need to be very persistent to obtain permanent care but don't give up. Sometimes it takes two or even three attempts.

YOU THE EXPERT

'Sometimes we just sat down and had a good laugh about something she'd done, like put her shoes in the fridge. When we laughed together, it helped a lot.' Ivy Tozer, Devizes

'He wet himself occasionally because he couldn't find the toilet. I painted the door red and he didn't have that problem again.' Ann McPherson, Solihull

44

Some people almost never visit their doctors – except when they are going on holiday and need travel immunisation and advice.

What's required? The situation is constantly changing and your GP's surgery should be up to date about what is required for different countries. Here are some of the main immunisations.

Tetanus, diptheria and polio Even though you were immunised as a child, you may need a booster to build up and maintain your immunity. These diseases are still very common throughout the world.

Hepatitis A and typhoid fever Advised if you're travelling to countries with poor sanitation and hygiene.

Cholera The vaccine is not very effective and so not recommended for most travellers

Hepatitis B Is only recommended if you are travelling or working for a long period abroad

Yellow fever Is serious and widespread in many Central and South American and African countries. Vaccine gives protection for ten years. A certificate may be required.

Depending on where you're going and what you're doing, you might also need immunisations against TB, meningitis, certain forms of encephalitis and rabies.

Malaria If you are going to a malaria zone, you will need to take anti-malaria tablets before, during and after your trip. But it's essential that you try and prevent yourself being bitten, by using mosquito nets at night, repellent, etc.

Remember, immunisations help but you should still be careful what you eat and drink and be scrupulous about hygiene

Leave yourself enough time Some immunisations – for instance, hepatitis B – require several injections and most take a little time to become fully effective. However, if you have to go away at short notice, it's still worth having your immunisations – any protection is better than none.

It's also preferable not to overload your body with too many immunisations at once.

What's the cost? Expect to be charged for immunisations required for travel. Some are quite expensive, but cheap in terms of the benefit you will get. Most are available in your local surgery, but you may have to go a specialist centre for the more unusual ones such as rabies.

Looking after yourself abroad
Standards of health and hygiene vary considerably from one country to another – take sensible precautions especially regarding food, water and other drinks, and exposure to the sun (see p.46)

develop – take folic acid supplements before you get pregnant.

There are three main types of skin cancer. Two are directly related to lifetime exposure to the sun so people in outdoor occupations are more at risk. They are fully curable and do not spread to other parts of the body. The third, melanoma is a very malignant form of cancer, which typically starts as a mole of altered shape and then rapidly spreads through the body.

Melanoma affects younger people and is thought to be related to intense exposure to sun that has caused sunburn – particularly in childhood.

Why do so many people now get melanoma? Partly because more people go abroad, but mainly because people expose themselves to the sun more. In the future, there may be more cases because of the reduction in the ozone level and the protection it offers from harmful radiation.

Danger from the sun – in Great Britain? Most people consider sun protection abroad, yet the sun in Britain is just as likely to cause damage. And beware spring sunshine – it might not seem hot, but because of ozone depletion as much UV radiation is getting through as would normally reach us in summer months – even in the north.

So what can I do to protect myself – slap on the sunscreen? Putting on sunscreens is important if there is no other way to protect yourself, but other measures should come first.

So what about sunscreens?

- choose one that is SPF 15 or above which protects against UVA and UVB
- apply liberally and re-apply it frequently
- be specially vigilant with children and keep babies out of the sun completely

Never let yourself get burnt

What's an SPF? It stands for sun protection factor. It's a measure of how long you can stay out in the sun without your skin becoming red – if you would normally get red in 10 minutes, an SPF15 sunscreen will allow you to stay out for 150 minutes. If you burn in less time, you can spend correspondingly less time in the sun. But this doesn't mean that you should aim to spend this much time in the sun.

YOU THE EXPERT

'Sunscreens don't work as well if stored at high temperatures – like in the glove box of the car – so I keep mine in the fridge, or in the cool box with the drinks on the beach.' Min Clough, Shepherds Bush

46

A jam doughnut contain

The most stressful thing about first aid is knowing what to do first. Here are the priorities.

- **don't panic**
- **ask for help** – shout for someone to call an ambulance or to assist you. If you are trained in life-saving techniques, use them,

but first

- **check for dangers to yourself** – and avoid becoming a second victim. Is there an electric hazard, gas, smoke or fumes, a danger of falling or being hit?
- **look for dangers to the injured person** and move them to safety, unless they have a possible back or neck injury in which case you should not move them unless absolutely necessary
- check for and treat immediate threats to life. Use the ABC of first aid
  - **airway** – is it clear? It may be blocked by the tongue or vomit – clear it if you can
  - **breathing** – use mouth to mouth resuscitation if the person isn't breathing
  - **circulation** – if there's no pulse, the heart has stopped. Use CPR (cardio-pulmonary resuscitation) by rhythmically pressing down on the chest to get the heart beating again
- if there is severe bleeding, attempt to stop it by pressing on the wound with a pad
- if the person is unconscious and has no obviously broken bones move them gently into the recovery position – as shown

TOP TIP

Mouth to mouth resuscitation and CPR are techniques requiring a degree of skill. If you watch Casualty, 999, or Baywatch, they will be very familiar to you. You may have also seen them in books. However, the only way to learn how to do them properly is to go on a course. There are many – run by the local British Red Cross and St John Ambulance whose number you will find in the phone book. They vary in length from a couple of hours to a few days.

Perhaps you've always wanted to do something like this.

Perhaps you've always put it off.

This time, just do it.

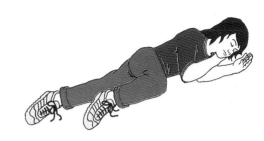

All the books listed here are the personal recommendations of the author. Most should be available in your library. The support groups listed offer a range of literature, information and advice. Since most of them are charities, a large SAE with your enquiry would be appreciated.

Medicines

BMA guide to prescription medicines and drugs Dorling Kindersley £12.99

Medicine, the self-help guide Penguin £6.95

Preparing for pregnancy

Planning a baby Dr Sarah Brewer Vermilion £8.99

Eating in pregnancy helpline 0114 242 4084
Advice on nutrition before, during and after pregnancy from experts

When pregnancy doesn't happen

Getting pregnant Prof. Robert Winston Pan £7.99

Becoming a mum

New pregnancy book HEA

Conception, pregnancy and birth Dr Miriam Stoppard Dorling Kindersley £16.95

National Childbirth Trust book of pregnancy birth and parenthood OUP £8.99

My child won't sleep Jo Douglas Penguin

Birth to five HEA

Your new baby Christine and Peter Hill Vermilion £8.99

Why they cry Hetty van Rijt & Frans Plooij Thorson's £9.99

CRY-SIS, BM Cry-sis,
London WC1N 3XX 0171 404 5011
Scotland 0131 334 5317

Association for Post-Natal Illness
0171 386 0868

Breastfeeding

NCT book of breastfeeding Mary Smale Vermilion £8.99

La Leche League, BM 3424, London WC1N 3XX 0171 242 1278

NCT, Alexandra House, Oldham Terrace, London W3 6NH 0181 992 8637

Weaning

Easy weaning Nanny knows best series Vermilion £4.99

Toddlers

Toddler taming Dr Christopher Green Vermilion £8.99
Wonderful, funny book which is a must for a family's sanity

Teenagers

Parent's guide to drugs and solvents D-mag drugs
Both these publications can be obtained by phoning D-COS on 01304 614 731

National drugs helpline 0800 77 66 00

Stress

British Association of Counsellors, 1 Regent Place, Rugby, Warks CV21 2PJ 01788 578328

The complete guide to stress management Dr Chandra Patel Vermilion £12.99

Lynn Marshall's instant stress cure Vermilion £8.99

Breast lumps and breast pain

Both the following books are excellent and cover cancer as well

The breast book Dr Miriam Stoppard Dorling Kindersley £14.99

Breast lumps J Smith & D Leaper Headway £5.99

Breast Cancer Care, 15/19 Britten St, London SW3 3TZ Info Line 0171 867 1103

Practical advice for women who have or fear they have, breast cancer

Imperial Cancer Research Fund, PO Box 123, London WC2A 3PX 0171 242 0200
Send a donation (min £1.50) for excellent *Breast cancer, saving more lives* booklet giving details of research, causes and treatment

Fashion targets breast cancer, breast health handbook Pandora £4.99 Brill!

The Breast Care Campaign, 1 St Mary Abbott's Place, London W8 6LS 0171 371 1510

Back pain

Beating back pain Dr J Tanner Dorling Kindersley £6.99
Very helpful, practical book on dealing with back pain

The National Back Pain Association, 16 Elmtree Road, Teddington, Middx TW11 8ST Send £2.50 plus large SAE for general information pack

For list of local practitioners contact British Chiropractic Association, 5 First Ave, Chelmsford, Essex, CM1 1RX 01245 353078

General Council of Osteopaths, 1–4 Suffolk St, London SW1Y 4HG 0181 839 2060

Chartered Society of Physiotherapy, 14 Bedford Row, London WC1R 4ED 0171 242 1941

The Health Education Authority publishes a wide range of leaflets on all aspects of health promotion – stopping smoking, healthy eating, physical activity, sensible drinking, and safer sex. They are available from local Health Promotion Units, which are often attached to hospitals and clinics. They are listed under Health Authority in the phone book. In case of difficulty contact HEA Customer Services, MBS, PO Box 269, Abingdon, Oxon. OX14 4YN